I HAVE A FRIEND WHO HAS MENTAL RETARDATION

HANNAH CARLSON, M.ED., CRC
DALE CARLSON

illustrated by
HOPE M. DOUGLAS, M.A.

CHANEY SHANNON PRESS
BICK PUBLISHING HOUSE
MADISON, CT

Text ©copyright 1995 by Hannah Carlson, M.Ed., CRC
and Dale Carlson
©illustrations 1995 by Hope M. Douglas, M.A.
©cover and book design 1995 by Jane Miller Productions

Edited by Ann Maurer

With thanks to Theodore Bromm of S.A.R.A.H., the Shoreline
Association of the Retarded and Handicapped

CHANEY SHANNON PRESS is a trademark of
BICK PUBLISHING HOUSE

Library of Congress Catalog Card Number: 95-79840

ISBN: 1-884158-09-9–Volume 3
ISBN: 1-884158-11-0–4 Volume Set

Printed by Royal Printing USA

Special needs/disabilities

"These books are an important service. They are informed, practical guides to feelings, behavior patterns, medical facts, technology, and resources for people who care about people with disabilities."
>–Richard Fucci, former president of the National Spinal
> Cord Injury Association

"Excellent, very informative."
>–Alan R. Ecker, M.D., Assistant Clinical Professor of
> Opthalmology, Yale University

"An invaluable source of help and comfort for friends and caregivers of people who have disabilities or special needs."
>–Mary Jon Edwards, Nationally Certified Therapeutic
> Horseback Riding Instructor, Special Olympics

"Excellent introductory handbooks about disabilities and special needs. They discuss medical conditions and rehabilitation, feelings and adaptive technology, and responsible attitudes both on the part of people with disabilities and people temporarily without them. The emphasis is on our common humanity, not our differences."
>–Lynn McCrystal, M.ED.,vice-president, The Kennedy Center

"The books offer professional information in an easy-to-use, uncomplicated style."
>–Renee Abbott, Group Home Director, S.A.R.A.H.,
> Shoreline Association for the Retarded and Handicapped

"Precise information, good reading for the layperson."
>–Jane Chamberlin, parent and employment supervisor, West
> Haven Community House

"Thank you for the opportunity to be a part of this work."
>–Christine M. Gaglio, employment specialist for the deaf, The
> Kennedy Center

CONTENTS

NOTE

Millions of people in the United States live with what are said to be disabilities. If you are family, caregiver, old friend or new friend to someone with an impaired ability, you are not alone. Learn that it is hard to live in a world so insistant on standing tall, being independent, and on regarding any handicap as a failure.

Friends of people with disabilities know that that their lives have not been significantly improved, despite attempts such as the Americans with Disabilities Act and the federal deinstitution-alization policy. Too often a social death precedes a physical one for people with disabilities such as mental retardation.

Understanding will lessen misconceptions and place the emphasis on abilities instead of disabilities, our common humani-ty, not our differences. There are resources for information, help, and reassurance to remind us that we are all in this together.

ACKNOWLEDGMENTS

Our gratitude to Theodore Harold Bromm and Renee Abbott, Group Home Director, both of S.A.R.A.H., the Shoreline Association of the Retarded and Handicapped; to Richard Fucci, former president of the National Spinal Cord Injury Association; to Alan Ecker, M.D., Assistant Clinical Professor of Opthalmology at Yale University; to Jane Chamberlin, parent and employment supervisor, West Haven Community House; and to Lynn McCrystal, M.Ed., vice-president, The Kennedy Center, for their counsel and editorial advice.

Our gratitude to Louis and Susan Weady, not only for Royal Printing, but for their guidance and patience with new editions, purchase orders, and shipping.

Our special thanks to Herb Swartz for his kindness and the use of his computers.

Our further special thanks to Danny Carlson for teaching us how to use computer capabilities for publishing.

And our thanks to Terrence Finnegan for providing Bick Publishing House with its own computer system.

1

MENTAL RETARDATION: CONDITIONS AND CAUSES

People can be born with mental retardation. Or they can acquire it during the course of their development through infancy, childhood, and adolescence; that is, before age 18. After age 18, people are given different diagnoses for the same symptoms, such as dementia or acquired brain injury.

Mental retardation is defined by the significant limitations someone has in functioning and adapting both to daily routines and new challenges during his or her life. IQ is a factor, but not the only one. Other factors include the ability to cope in the following areas: self-care, home living, communication social skills, community use, leisure health and safety, self-direction, functional academics, work.

CONDITIONS

Self-care and home living

People with mental retardation may have difficulty dressing or feeding themselves, and/or washing or toileting themselves. At home, they may struggle with cooking, cleaning, shopping for food, and keeping their homes in good condition. Some are profoundly unable to complete any of these functions on their own, and need total care and supervision.

Communication

Many people with mental retardation have significant difficulty in understanding your thoughts and feelings and expressing their own. They may not be able to use the gestures, vocal tones, and facial expressions other people use that help to interpret messages and convey ideas. Some people with mental retardation can not read or write.

This does not mean that these individuals do not have thoughts or feelings. All people think about their lives and have reactions to their experiences, positive and negative. All people feel excited or anxious sometimes, sad and lonely at other times.

Social skills, community use, leisure

Many people with mental retardation have very limited abilities to make friends, go out into their neighborhoods, or participate in recreational activities with others.

This limitation may be more a function of exclusion, of other people not wanting to be around those with mental retardation. They do not, therefore, get to participate in social events or leisure activities in the community, sometimes even just go to the movies. Often, they do not get to experience friendships or even the most ordinary of social exchanges.

Health and safety, self-direction

Some people with mental retardation do not show the judgement and decision making skills essential in staying healthy and safe. They may not understand the application of such rules as looking both ways when crossing a street, wearing a coat in cold weather, wearing a seatbelt, or not talking to strangers.

More important, they may also not know how to speak up for themselves, advocate for their own rights or protection, or seek assistance when they need it. This limitation leaves many people with mental retardation potentially vulnerable to others who might take advantage of, neglect, or abuse them.

Functional academics

Although some individuals with mental retardation attend regular (mainstream) elementary and high schools, others need special help in learning basic concepts required for later in life and attend special education classes or schools that offer specialized teaching.

Examples: classes in awareness of the physical environment (instead of science class, health class, and sex education); money management (instead of math class); and symbol recognition and symbol use which may include reading and writing (instead of English class).

Work

Some people with mental retardation require special assistance in order to get and keep jobs. They may get vocational training to learn work skills and behaviors, time awareness and management, and travel training to get to work. While on the job, some individuals need ongoing support from a job coach to help them apply the skills they learned.

Going to a special school does not mean people with mental

retardation cannot learn. It means they benefit from special supports while learning to help themsleves get what they need from the lesson. While at work, having a job coach does not mean people with mental retardation cannot learn or perform a job. In fact, studies have shown that these individuals show more dedication to their jobs through lower absenteeism. They also produce more consistent levels of work over time than their nondisabled counterparts.

CAUSES OF MENTAL RETARDATION

People are born with mental retardation or acquire mental retardation in a variety of ways. Physical disorders or syndromes may accompany mental retardation. These disorders can inhibit peoples' abilities to control their reflexes or other parts of their nervous systems. They can affect bone and muscle development. These disorders can cause defects information and function of organs. They can do the same to spine and brain development and function.

Here is a partial list of disorders associated with mental retardation. The causes of mental retardation are divided in three categories: prenatal, perinatal, and postnatal.

Prenatal (during pregnancy)

1. chromosomal disorders: Down syndrome and x-linked gene syndromes (Fragil X syndrome, Turner syndrome, and Klinefelter syndrome)

2. syndrome disorders which include;

a) neurocutaneous disorders (Louis-Bar, Basil cell nevus, and

Tuberous slerosis)

- b)muscular disorders(Becker, Congential,Duchenne, and Myotonic muscular dystrophies)
- c)*ocular disorders* (Norrie syndrome, Aniridia-Wilm's tumor syndrome, and Lowe syndrome)
- d)craniofacial disorders(Acrocephaly-cleftlip-radial aplasia syndrome and Carpenter syndrome)
- e)skeletal disorders (Hypochondroplasia, Acrodysostosis)

3. inborn metabolic disorders involving amino acids (Phenylketonuria), carbohydrates, urea cycle disorders, and nucleac acid disorders

4. developmental disorders of brain formation(spina bifida and Hydrocephalus)

5. environmental influences (malnutrition, toxins, drugs, maternal diseases)

Perinatal (in and around labor and delivery)

1. intrauterine disorders: acute placental insufficiency, abnormal labor and delivery, and multiple gestation

2. neonatal disorders: intracranial hemorrhage, neonatal seizures, respiratory disorders; infections – Meningitis, Rubella, Syphilis, Toxoplasmosis; head trauma at birth; nutritional disorders; metabolic disorders – Hypothyroidism, Hypoglycemia

Postnatal (after delivery)

1. head injuries (accidents, abuse)
2. infections (Encephilitis and Meningitis)

10

3. demyelinating disorders (Encephalomyelitis)
4. degenerative disorders (Rett syndrome, Parkinson's
   Disease and Huntington's Disease— juvenile type)
5. seizure disorders
6. toxic metabolic disorders
7. malnutrition
8. environmental deprivation
9. hypoconnection syndrome

IMPROVE THE ENVIRONMENT, IMPROVE THEIR ABILITIES

Many people diagnosed with mental retardation show significant improvements in their abilities to function and adapt in their lives and work, if provided a healthy, supportive, stimulating home and community life. In other words, you and I can make a significant impact on strengthening the skills and quality of functioning of a person with mental retardation with the type and amount of assistance and care we are willing to share.

Remember that we are all to some extent emotionally immature, frequently wrong, and often cruel. It might be as well to question who has the mental disability?

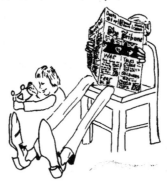

2

THEIR FEELINGS, YOUR FEELINGS

While there are many myths about people with mental retardation, the truth is that they have feelings and emotional needs just as all people do. Like others, many people with mental retardation are sensitive to how they are perceived by others and want very much to be included and accepted by those around them.

THEIR FEELINGS

1. They are sensitive to the environment and are aware if they are safe and accepted.
2. They are subject to low self-esteem when others treat them in demeaning, abusive, or neglectful ways.
3. They like to go to the same movies, sporting events, restaurants, art exhibits, concerts that all people do.
4. They are attracted to many of the same qualities nondisabled people are in others: friendliness, loyalty, respect, good humor. It is important to distinguish: mental retardation is not a mental illness. Those with mental retardation are subject to the same mental illnesses as other people including depression, anxiety, schizophrenia, and adjustment disorders from childhood or adult traumatic experiences.

Sadly, children and adults with disabilities such as mental

retardation are more vulnerable to abuse and neglect from others. Therefore, there may be a greater likelihood of people with mental retardation who experience adjustment disorders as result.

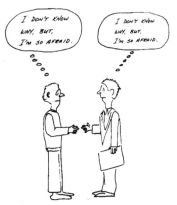

YOUR FEELINGS

1. **anxiety:** I don't know why, but I am afraid

I don't know how to behave

I don't know if he or she understands me

He or she is acting too friendly

I don't know what to do or say

I don't understand what he or she is saying

I will probably say or do the wrong thing

2. **disgust:** I don't like to see the physical conditions of this disability; possible malformations of someone's face, mouth, head, body ,or limbs.

I don't like to witness their lack of control over their own bodies: shaking; tics; spasms.

3. **fear:** I could get it

They may get aggressive

They may have a seizure

4. **compassion:** Their lives must be difficult

I want to help

5. **enjoyment:** This person is a lot of fun to be around

Knowing this person adds more to my life

Clearly, there are as many possible feelings as there are people who have them. These feelings are likely to vary depending on the extent to which the person's disability impacts on your experience. For example, if the two of you are strangers waiting for a bus, you may experience no more than idle curiosity. However, if you are spending eight or more hours a day with someone because he or she is your co-worker, you may have more responses. Studies have shown that the more experiences people share with others who have mental retardation, the more everybody feels acceptance, comfort, and pleasure.

3

MANNERS THAT MATTER: BOTH SIDES

A similar interest or a shared activity can bring people into the lives of those with disabilities. Most often, people without disabilities come to help those with disabilities. They can be paid workers such as a job coach or residential counselor; volunteer workers such as those in recreational programs; or a co-worker or stranger who just steps in at the moment of a problem.

In these cases, the disability becomes the focus, not the person. The symptoms or limitations of the disability become the point instead of what is really important – the opportunity for friendship.

You will want to be aware of what you think, say, and do. When you are helping someone with mental retardation and/or developing a friendship, understanding is essential. Understanding means listening and caring; not for what you expect the person to say, but for what he or she is really feeling or thinking.

YOUR MANNERS
General behavior
1. Remember that someone is a person with a disability, not a disabled person.
2. Focus on what the person can do, and offer assistance only where it is obviously needed.

3. Allow extra time for the other person to interpret what you say, or to perform an activity, if he or she needs it.

4. Treat adults with mental retardation as adults, not children. Don't drag them around. Show them the respect another adult deserves when speaking to them or about them to others. For example, do not refer to an adult as a "good boy or girl."

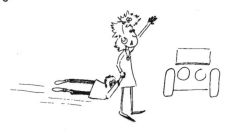

5. Remember, we all have handicaps. Some are more visible than others. Some can be hidden, some cannot.

Communicating

1. Look at people with mental retardation and establish eye contact when you speak to them.

2. Speak directly to them, not about them.

3. Speak calmly, clearly, and slowly. It is not necessary (or polite) to shout or overexaggerate your words.

4. Use gestures, pictures, and facial expressions to help the other person understand you.

5. Listen closely to the person who may have difficulty articulating words. Do not pretend to understand what you do not.

6. Be prepared to repeat your sentence. Feel free to ask them to repeat theirs.

7. Learn a few signs in American Sign Language. It is easy and fun. It is the language many people with mental retardation use to communicate.

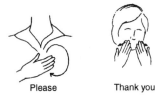

Please   Thank you

8. If you do not understand the message after trying the different ways   recommended here, it is acceptable to ask for assistance from someone who is accompanying the person.

THEIR MANNERS

1. Allow extra time for people without disabilities to understand you. They are not used to your way of talking or gesturing.
2. Be prepared to repeat what you said. Ask them to repeat what they say, if you don't understand them.
3. Speak calmly, clearly, and slowly. It is not necessary (nor

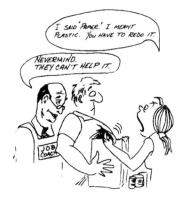

17

polite) to shout or overexaggerate your words.

4. Use gestures, pictures, facial expressions, or write down what you want, if they do not understand you.

5. Teach them some signs in sign language. Remember, they can learn, too.

GETTING TO KNOW YOU

When getting to know someone with mental retardation, ask the same questions asked when getting to know anyone.

Ask about:

- favorite stores at the mall
- favorite movies
- favorite foods
- favorite activities
- kind of work, types of tasks done at work or day program
- likes and dislikes about work, friends, homelife

It is everybody's responsibility

It is up to all of us, with or without disabilities, to interrupt the ignorance, prejudice, and indifference we encounter in our everyday lives. In order to change old systems or ways of thinking, we need to step in and speak up.

Education is the weapon of choice. Use your knowledge to inform others to think about the abilities of people with mental retardation, not their limitations. That they have thoughts and feelings just as all people do. That there are specific ways available to communicate with people with mental retardation such as the ways discussed in this chapter. That our caring and involvement with people with mental retardation can and does make a significant contribution to their lives and ours.

Take a class in sign language with a friend. It is a lot of fun. And it can be quite useful in loud environments or places where you don't want others to know what you are saying.

Use ASL as a way of including everyone in our multicultural world: this would be a significant step in acknowledging people with special needs as part of our community, and not outside of it.

4

SEEKING DIAGNOSIS

Some people with mental retardation spend their entire lives without ever being diagnosed. They graduate from high school and get jobs. They get married and have children.

Most people are diagnosed when they are children. During the course of their development, their performance falls below the accepted ranges of skill development. Their parents and teachers usually notice that they are not developing at the same rate as other children. Their pediatricians refer them to specialists for testing.

A diagnosis of mental retardation is determined by a person meeting specific criteria in the following three areas: intellectual functioning level; adaptive skill level; and age of onset. Age of onset is important. To be classified as having mental retardation, a person must be under the age of 18.

INTELLECTUAL FUNCTIONING LEVEL: I.Q.

Using one's intelligence quotient (I.Q.) is one of the oldest means of determining mental retardation. The most common tests administered include the Stanford-Binet Intelligence Scale, the Wechsler Intelligence Scale for Children-III, Weschler Adult Intelligence Scale-Revised, the Weschler Preschool and Primary

Scale of Intelligence, and the Kaufman Assessment Battery for Children.

A score of 100 is considered average intelligence. Intelligence tests allow for a 15 point deviation (1 standard deviation) of this score in order to stay within the average range. That means an I.Q. score of 85 to 115 is within the range of average intelligence.

An I.Q. score of 70-75 is considered significant for mental retardation. That means, the person scored approximately 2 standard deviations away from the average score.

Scores below 70-75 are used to indicate levels of mental retardation such as moderate, severe, and profound. However, these tests only provide a score. They can not supply necessary information about how the intellectual limitations affect the person's ability to negotiate the demands of living and working.

More current approaches are moving away from such harsh and useless labels. Today, the focus is on levels of functioning or adaptive skills, and to identify what level of support is needed for each individual.

ADAPTIVE SKILLS LEVEL

Adaptive skills level is the assessment of a person's ability to function in the environment, solve problems, make decisions, and develop relationships with others.

The adaptive skills level measures the functioning levels described in chapter one:

      a) self-care, home living, communication

      b) social skills, community use, leisure

c) health and safety, self-direction

d) functional academics

e) work

Prefered tests for assessing adaptive skills levels include: AAMD Adaptive Behavior Scales (ABS); the School Edition of the ABS; the revised Vineland Adaptive Behavior Scales; the Scales of Independent Behavior; and the Comprehensive Test of Adaptive Behavior.

ABILITIES AND SUPPORT NEEDS

This is where to keep the focus – on abilities and support needs!

Identifying the strengths and weaknesses in coping with the demands of daily life, school, and work, is more useful than simply measuring I.Q. Adaptive skills assessments also indicate the type and extent of assistance needed in order for the person to perform more independently or successfully.

Levels of assistance are identified as follows:

1. Intermittent: short term, on an as-needed-basis. Support may be periodic, such as when someone loses a job or relocates to a new neighborhood. Extent of support may be intense, although time-limited.

2. Limited: support may not be as intense as intermittent support and is defined by its consistency over time (such as transitional help in learning a new job or bus route to school or work).

3. Extensive: support is not time-limited and provides for regular involvement at home or work. An example of this is the presence of an attendant at the   person's home when he or she returns from work to settle them in and assist with making dinner.

4. Pervasive: support is long-term, consistent and   intense. The nature of the support may be life-sustaining and can include work and home settings (such as the need for a personal care attendent for dressing, feeding, toileting, traveling, etc).

Choosing a support system

Once a person has been diagnosed with mental retardation, he or she becomes eligible under various Federal and state laws for special services. A support system is developed to coordinate and provide the services for someone who has mental retardation.

A good system for support will focus on the individual's:

a) personality, their likes and dislikes

b) functional level, their skills and weaknesses

c) already existing and available supports such as family
     members and friends.

In general

People have different styles of interacting with others and varying abilities in coping with the demands of living in this world. The same is true with people who have mental retardation.   Therefore, in selecting professionals, schools, programs, and group homes it is essential to keep the individual at the center of the plan or system. This is referred to as "person-centered planning" in the service field of mental retardation.

DOCTORS

Medical support

Medical treatment, surgery, physical, occupational and/or speech therapy. For those born with accompanying medical conditions such as arm or leg deformities or weaknesses, speech or hearing problems, therapy can begin while they are infants in order to correct the condition or minimize the impact of the physical disabilities on later functioning.

Empathy

When choosing doctors, look for empathy, knowledge of the disabilities involved, and the doctor's ability to assist you in accessing additional community resources.

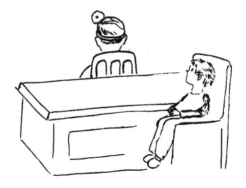

Empathy is nicer.

SCHOOLS

Educational support

Individual educational plans are developed for each person, identifying strengths and weaknesses. Good plans recommend specific goals and objectives which address the educational needs.

Mainstream education

Some children with mental retardation are able to meet the challenges of a regular school environment if provided extra support. Plans for these students usually include one-on-one tutoring and/or having a special education paraprofessional in a mainstream classroom to work individually with the student. Some special education classes are held within the school. These students are able to develop friendships with other children who do not have disabilities. In order to receive other services, they may have to leave school early each day to go to a separate therapy service.

Special education

Other children, who would find it too overwhelming in a mainstream school, or overstimulating in a regular classroom, are educated in special education schools. There, the curriculum focuses on more basic lessons and developing practical skills needed in everyday life. They develop social relationships with other students with similar disabilities who attend the school. They are able to receive all their services or therapies in one location.

When choosing a school, you may wish to investigate the staffs' philosophies toward the role of education, community integration, and quality of life for children with disabilities such as mental retardation. Compare their views with yours regarding the kind of adults these children will become: how they will fit into society, live, and work.

If you have a preference, research and compare the degree

to which the school emphasizes vocational training vs. basic academics; signing vs lip reading/speaking; and where their students go after graduation: vocational training; day programs; or out on their own to obtain jobs and integrate into their own neighborhoods. The best schools will design person-centered plans which take into account individual preferences, strengths, and outside supports (family, friends, other social services).

Transportation needs, residential programs

It is also recommended that you research the school's standing on service delivery and quality with the regional Board of Education. If the school has a residential program, check with the licensing state agency for mental retardation services to insure they are up to date with their inspections and compliance measures.

WORK

Vocational training

Job training and placement programs are available for adults with mental retardation (usually beginning around the age of 21). Adults are trained to perform jobs in areas such as:

- grocery bagging
- retail (ticketing, clothes hanging, receiving, and recovery)
- mailroom work
- custodial work
- recycling
- food services (food preparation, busing, and dishwashing)
- clerical work (filing, photocopying, collating)

• assembly and packaging work

They obtain jobs with the assistance of the placement program and receive the support of a job coach to learn the job, work schedule, and transportation route to the job.

Vocational training

When choosing a vocational program, it is important to consider the philosophies of the staff who will be working with the adult in the program. And to compare their points of view with yours as when choosing a school. In the case of a vocational program, however, it is very important to learn where the participants get jobs, what kinds of jobs, how much available support there is to assist the adult who is entering the program, and in general, how long the support is available. Program descriptions, program evaluation reports, and placement statistics are good sources for this information. These should be made available to you, upon request. Also, ask for other program participants' names and phone numbers so that you may ask them their opinion about the services the program provides.

Good vocational programs will be accredited by national organizations such as CARF (Commission on Accreditation for Rehabilitation Facilities) or JCAHO (Joint Commission on Accreditation of Healthcare Organizations).

LIVING ARRANGEMENTS
Residential support

Some people with mental retardation live on their own or

with their families. They may or may not need some level of support from family and friends in order to conduct their daily lives, do their laundry, shopping, and banking.

Group homes

Many people with mental retardation live in group homes or supported living arrangements. House managers and residential counselors provide whatever level of support is necessary to assist the residents achieve the highest level of independence possible. Residents participate in shopping, cleaning their homes, caring for themselves, and going out into the community to see movies or visit museums.

When choosing a group home or supported living arrangement, again, compare the philosophy of the program to your own. You may also want to compare their house rules to the customs of the adult who is moving in. Consider any changes the adult will need to make in terms of how he or she currently lives.

Areas to consider:

- recreational activities and how they are scheduled
- dietary menus
- means of transportation
- type of neighborhood (urban vs. rural)
- noise level of house mates
- number and sex of house mates
- any unacceptable behaviors such as aggression or stealing on the part of housemates and how they are addressed

Good residential programs should be licensed by a state agency for mental retardation.

Some people with mental retardation live in large facilities such as state institutions or Intermediate Care Facilities (ICF's). They may or may not be able to care for themselves. Those who are independent in caring for themselves and/or can perform work, may go out to work and return in the afternoon.

Those who require extensive supports, may attend a day program focused on activities that engage their interest during the day. Or, they may remain in their facilities with no program at all.

Of course, institutional care is an unacceptable way to live and be treated. Qualitative progress in this area of service delivery is slow to happen and remains an issue of contention for service providers in this field. However, many states are closing their larger institutions, and transfering the residents to private service providers who can better meet the individual needs of each person.

5

LIVING WITH MENTAL RETARDATION
A DAY IN A LIFE

In the 16th century, people born with mental retardation were treated as freaks or delinquents. They were left to die, used as court jesters, or punished for having been born with this disorder.

During the next several hundred years, asylums were constructed to house certain people away from the rest of the community. Residents of the asylums included beggars, active alcoholics and drug addicts, the homeless, prostitutes, and people with disabilities such as mental retardation. The carryovers from these asylums are the large state-owned institutions of today.

Conditions have been improving for individuals with mental retardation. Many large institutions are closing. Smaller, privately-owned service providers have opened group homes to replace the institutions. Perceptions have improved from the early 1900's when names such as "moron" and "imbecile" were used to classify those with mental retardation. Today, those terms are considered offensive.

In 1990, the Americans with Disabilities Act was passed as a Federal Civil Rights Law. It provides for equal opportunity, full participation, independent living, and self-sufficiency for all people with disabilities in employment and life. The law has already helped many people achieve access to jobs, housing, public buildings (such as clinics, voting booths, schools, and churches), and transportation that were previously inaccessible or unattainable. For example, previous to this law supporting accessibility, many people with physical disabilities could not vote, worship religion within their churches or temples, or attend schools, because they could not gain entrance to the buildings.

While the law can mandate and enforce regulations concerning accessibility and policy, it can not institute a change in peoples' attitudes. In this area, people with disabilities still struggle for the right to be treated equally and with dignity.

MEGAN

Megan lives in a group home with men and women who work in the community. This morning Megan overslept. She missed her turn on the schedule to take a shower. She grabs whatever few minutes she can to brush her teeth and comb her hair. Megan worries that people at work will know she didn't shower. She puts on her clothes.

In the next room, Megan can hear shouting again. John often keeps the others up at night with his tantrums. It makes Megan anxious to hear all the yelling. Last night, Megan got very little sleep because of John's yelling. Megan can hear a staff person trying to talk to John.

Megan runs to the bus stop down the block. The bus is already there. She is afraid she will miss it and be late for work.

Her boss will be mad at her.

Megan makes the bus just before it pulls away from the curb. Making her way to the back, trying to catch her breath, Megan overhears one woman say to the other, "The mentally retarded are so lucky. They live in their own little worlds. Nothing ever bothers them. They are always so happy."

MARK

Mark is 45 years old and has mental retardation. At present, he lives in a group home with five other adults. At dinner, Mark hoards his food even though he is free to eat whenever and how much he pleases. Mark tends to rock in his chair and hum to himself when not engaged in work or other activities. To others, his behavior may seem strange, asocial, or without cause. To Mark, his behavior is how he copes with the world as he experiences it.

When he was 7, his family, on the advice of their physicians, placed him in a state institution. While growing up, Mark was exposed to the intermittent neglect and abuse that is common in such facilities. As a result, Mark developed certain behaviors as a way of coping with his vulnerability to these conditions.

Mark learned to hoard food to ward off hunger, since he was unprotected by staff when others took his food. Sometimes, Mark was not given enough to eat. Sometimes he was not fed at all.

Mark rocked back and forth when he got anxious. It soothed him, since he received little, if any, affection. Mark's humming served to tune out the loud noises such as others' yelling. It also kept him company and provided stimulation in the long hours he spent alone, without anything to occupy his mind.

At age 40, Mark was removed from the institution and placed in the group home and vocational program. Although Mark, his family, and the institution all believed he would never walk, it was found that his inability to walk was based on the shoes with which he had been provided. He had never been provided with proper shoes, and the improper ones had deformed his feet. Orthopedic shoes now enable Mark to walk independently to work. He is one of the most productive workers at his job and has established warm relationships with his co-workers.

KEVIN

Kevin is 27 years old. Kevin has cerebral palsy and mental retardation. He lives in a group home and is cared for by staff especially trained to assist him in bathing, dressing, eating, getting around, and performing different activities. He spends almost all of his waking day in a wheelchair. Although he cannot speak, Kevin communicates with others by answering "yes" and "no" questions with his eyebrows and eyes. When first meeting Kevin, people

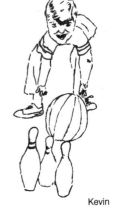

Kevin

33

learn how to understand him, and how to use his preferred method of communication: that is, to use "yes" and "no" questions.

Like Mark, Kevin spent his childhood in an institution. Due to severe neglect and malnutrition, Kevin did not grow to his proper height. He developed cystic fibrosis. He was never trained to develop his capacities for work or independence until he was placed in a private group home as an adult.

Today, Kevin enjoys his participation in a horticultural day program. He spends his weekends out shopping and going to visit friends in other group homes. He is a member of the Special Olympics and competes in local bowling and track games.

LISA

Lisa is 30 years old. She has Down syndrome and lives with her mother. Lisa holds a part time job and is assisted by a job coach to transport her to the job and supervise her during the day. Lisa is a good worker and very friendly, making her one of the most popular employees at the company. On her birthday, the employees provided her with a surprise birthday party and presents.

When Lisa was a child, her mother fought the physician's recommendation and decided against placing Lisa in an institution. Lisa grew up at home and attended a special education school. Her mother and siblings had to assist Lisa in learning how to care for herself. They also had to defend Lisa's right to be a citizen in the community like anyone else. Lisa was exposed to people staring, ridiculing, or avoiding contact with her.

Having Down syndrome means Lisa looks different than most other people. She has lower set ears, wider set eyes, and a stockier build than others. She does not learn as quickly as some.

Being a human being means Lisa has the same feelings as others and enjoys many of the same experiences; she likes to laugh, be accepted, and feel proud of her achievements.

A NOTE ABOUT FAMILIES

Having a child with mental retardation requires parents and siblings to examine and, perhaps significantly adjust their values and expectations about mental retardation and their child who has it. It means special services, special schools. It may also include special medical attention if the child is born with other physical conditions (congenital heart disorders, kidney or liver disorders, hearing or vision impairments, dental problems, etc). Entire family structures are altered; finances can be drained.

As the child develops, family members must adapt their ways of living to meet the developmental pace of the child. Parents are not just parents anymore. They are guardians, advocates, and, sometimes, activists for their childrens' rights to receive adequate care and equal opportunity. Siblings must adjust to receiving less attention and perhaps greater responsibilities within the household or in protecting their brother or sister with mental retardation when out in the neighborhood.

Even into adulthood, the person with mental retardation may

require continued support and advocacy from his or her family. Many family members continue acting as guardians, making decisions about medical treatment, finances, and where their loved one will live and work.

It should be noted, some families become too exhausted or too old to continue this amount of care. Some families have neither the ability nor the desire to perform such caretaking for their child. In such cases, guardians are appointed for them by the state.

To have a family member with mental retardation can be very rewarding: it can deepen bonds and make relationships more meaningful and appreciated. But, it can also drive apart families who can not meet the many challenges mental retardation can present. The first shock and grief experienced by parents at first learning that a child has been born with Down syndrome, or any other mental disability, can turn to hope and joy as they learn that in many ways their child is no different than any other child, that their child has the same fun at the movies, the same pleasure in throwing a ball with pals or dad, the same capacity for affection, for work, for living life.

But the insensitivity of the best-meaning people, the ignorance about the many capabilities and great potential and deepest feelings of those born with a disability is heart-breaking. And despite the Individuals with Disabilities Education Act that guarantees an access to educational, employment, housing, and recreational opportunities, there continue to be those who belittle and exclude.

And there is the worry about the future. Where will my child live when he or she grows up? Who will take care of my child when I'm gone? Will there be friends who care and understand and guide my child toward a life full of possibilities instead of closed doors, barred gates?

More is needed for all of us than just a place to eat and sleep. Billy Golfus, hemiplegic, is a film journalist. He says: " Being disabled is as close as you can get to being invisisble. It makes people with disabilities angry, being treated as sick and unable and without a future. What makes you think being disabled is suffering? It's other people's attitudes that makes us suffer."

6

RESOURCES; TRAINING; JOB OPPORTUNITIES; HOUSING;
TRANSPORTATION; FUNDING; APPLIANCES;
DIET AND EXERCISE

For those who know about the systems of social services and how to navigate through them, resources are usually accessible. For the rest of us, we will require a map to find the services, a directory to know who to talk to, and a translator to explain to us in normal language what the procedures and conditions are for obtaining the assistance we need.

WRITE IT DOWN

It is important to keep notes on every conversation when talking to any social service agency.

Always write down:

- the date and time of contact
- whether it was in person or on the phone
- phone number (and extension)
- name and title of the person with whom you talked
- stated agreements or conditions for receiving services
- dates to follow-up on stated agreements or conditions

Having this information on record can mean the difference between the social service agency providing what was agreed to in the conversation and denying any record of your approaching the agency at all.

38

BE PERSISTENT AND POLITE

The old phrase, "the squeaky wheel gets the oil" applies here. Do not give in or give up, but remember that the person you are talking to has the service or information you need. Acknowledge that you do not know the systems as well as the person you are talking to. Ask for help and assistance wherever you need it.

SOCIAL SERVICE RESOURCES

Contact the local or regional division of the State Department of Mental Retardation and Department of Social Services. Phone numbers can be located in the government section of any phone book. They will arrange an appointment with you and the person you are referring. Once the person is found eligible, they will be able to provide the best social, educational, or job training programs available in your area.

Children

Children with mental retardation are provided services through the town's or city's Board of Education. They are automatically eligible with a diagnosis of mental retardation to receive whatever special services they require due to Public Laws such as the Education for All Handicapped Children Act passed in 1975. The Board of Education is required to ensure services are provided. You will need to investigate and possibly advocate to ensure the services provide the quality of care or support for your child.

Agencies that advocate for rights

There are a variety of not-for-profit agencies established to assist people with mental retardation or other disabilities to advocate for their rights, jobs, transportation, housing, energy and food assistance, protection against abuse, and legal issues. Eligibility for the services are usually based on financial need. The Department of Mental Retardation may have the names and phone numbers for these agencies. They should be listed in the phone book. The local Chamber of Commerce should have published lists of the agencies.

FUNDING

The Department of Mental Retardation, Department of Social Services (through PASS, Plan for Achieving Self Sufficiency), and state vocational rehabilitation services all provide funding for vocational training and job placement. Other services are also sponsored by these departments. Each organization should be able to provide a list of all the services they sponsor.

TRANSPORTATION

If public transportation is not available or not accessible, traveling independently is very difficult, maybe impossible. Some cities and towns have established transportation services for those who require special assistance. However, the services are unreliable at best. People need to call constantly, even if they have purchased a subscription service for regular rides (such as going to work). It is important to leave time for a late van. Many people using the service need to arrange a pick up 30 to 60 minutes before they would normally leave to travel to work.

LOW AND HIGH TECH AIDS

There are assistive devices, equipment, tools, or gadgets to make any task easier to accomplish for a person with a disability. Many low technology aids are commonly used in non-disabled homes:

- electric can and bottle openers
- Lazy Susans
- "clappers" (noise activated electronic appliances)
- "talking" or beeping clocks and watches
- electronic phone books
- slide bar light switches
- speaker phones
- remote controls
- "mouse" cursor guide used with computers
- single arm water faucet controls
- hand-held shower heads
- anything involving a velcro attachment

Other low tech items include such small rubber mats to prevent slipping, raised edged plates, and cutting boards with nails to hold the food in place. Grab bars and wheelchairs can be purchased through catalogs or a pharmacy that supplies medical equipment.

High technology aids can include computer operated equipment such as communication boards and motorized wheelchairs, as well as Telecommunication Devices for the Deaf (TDD's) which are used for phone communication for those with hearing and/or speech impairments.

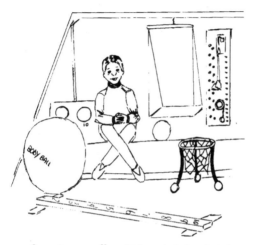

Sometimes staff could be a little less helpful.

DIET AND EXERCISE

All people benefit from following a healthy diet and getting regular exercise. Some people with mental retardation have slower than usual metabolism rates or medications that promote easier weight gain. For these people, special diet plans are necessary.

Also for these people, exercise is particularly important in order not to complicate their health with obesity that can lead to adult diabetes, cardiovascular disorders, or heart disease.

Special Olympics

The Special Olympics was originally developed from a day-care camp for people with mental retardation started by Eunice Kennedy Shriver. It served children and adults, offering them opportunities to participate in sports. The Kennedy Foundation later turned this camp into a national chain of camps.

In 1968, Mrs. Shriver established the International Special Olympics Games. The competitions took place at Soldiers' Field in Chicago with approximately 1000 athletes.

Today, the International Special Olympics comprises over 22 sports, in 75 countries with over 1,000,000 athletes. Events occur year round. People participate at all levels of ability. Each state offers local and area competitions. Athletes go on to compete at national and international levels. In the summer of 1995, for instance, Connecticut hosted the International Special Olympics.

The Special Olympics is comprised of volunteers who assist the athletes at all levels of competition. All the coordinators, coaches, bus or van drivers, referrees, medical professionals, and cheerleaders are volunteers. To volunteer, simply contact the International Headquarters to find the state or local office nearest you. The International Headquarter's address and phone number can be found in the appendix, sources for help.

7

FIX YOUR ATTITUDE AND YOUR HOUSE

The Americans with Disabilities Act (ADA) does not apply to lives and homes of private citizens. However, making your home and activities accessible to those with disabilities is an effective step toward including people with disabilities in your life. Some people with mental retardation have physical limitations as well. "Reasonable accomodation," according to the ADA, "means making adjustments to architectural and procedural barriers that are readily achievable."

TEST YOURSELF: AN EXPERIMENT IN NEW PERCEPTIONS

Look closely at your living room, bedroom, bathroom, and kitchen. Ask yourself how you access the things that you need to use. Now, put a chair in the middle of the room. Ask yourself how you would access the same things from your seated position, as if you were in a wheelchair.

Making your living environment more accessible may mean adjusting furniture to make it easier for those with a cane, crutch, or wheelchair to pass through. It may mean setting up lower shelves.

When you are out in the community, shopping or eating at a restaurant, try the exercise you did at home. One important step toward making your community more accessible would be to encourage the store or restaurant owners to make "reasonable accomodations" that are "readily achievable" just as you have done at home. Remind them that people with disabilities are customers, too.

CHANGE THE ENVIRONMENT

In changing environments to include people with disabilities, we will change attitudes as well. We can support some people with physical assistance. Others rely on our judgement for safety. It is up to us to make the environment accessible and safe for all people.

It is up to all of us to include all of us.

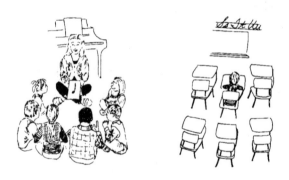

8

SELECTED DISORDERS

DOWN SYNDROME

Down syndrome is a chromosomal disorder. Many individuals are trisomic for chromosome number 21. That means, they have 47 chromosomes instead of 46. Physical features include: vertical folds covering the inner part of the eye from the root of the nose to the inside tip of the eyebrow; slanted or diagonally shaped eyes; broad bridge of the nose, protruding tongue, open mouth, square-shaped ears, diminished muscle tone, and, possibly, congenital heart disease. People with Down syndrome have different degrees of mental retardation.

AUTISM

Considered a psychomotor deficit, autism affects the ability to process information when interacting with people, communicating, and reacting to the environment. Individuals with autism show preferences for isolation, indifference towards others, and significant difficulty integrating and following rules of conduct that are socially expected and accepted. People with autism have great difficulty in communicating. Some never develop verbal language.

In addition, those with autism display a limited range of behaviors or movements that are repetitive and restricted in character: arm flapping; hand posturing; grimacing; or unusual gait patterns. They can appear hypersensitive to some sensations or experiences such as tastes and sounds, while totally unresponsive to others such as pain.

More than 1/2 of all those diagnosed with autism also have mental retardation.

Some people with autism have specific talents in areas of music, visual arts, mechanics, math, and mnemonic skills (calendar calculations). People with an ability in one of these areas are able to perform tasks with amazing precision and accuracy. Some people can play highly complex music they have heard only once. Others are able to calculate the day of the week of any date in the future or the day of the week a person was born given the birth date and year. These abilities are associated with the right side of the brain functioning and are called Savant syndromes.

CEREBRAL PALSY

Cerebral palsy can occur at birth or during early infancy. Muscles are uncoordinated, spastic, weak, or even paralyzed. While cerebral palsy is nonprogressive, it can be accompanied by seizures, behavioral disorders, learning disorders, and mental retardation. Physical therapy, occupational therapy, speech therapy, and surgery are usually prescribed to repair or strengthen weakened or deformed limbs, or to improve muscle function and coordination.

SOURCES FOR HELP

1. American Association on Mental Retardation
   444 North Capitol Street, NW, Suite 846
   Washington, DC 20001-1512
   800-424-3688

AAMR provides education and advocacy through research, publications, and conferences. It can provide information on additional resources for local areas, nationwide. Memberships are welcome and come with a monthly journal and listings for recent publications.

2. Office of Disability
   Social Security Administration
   Department of Health and Human Services
   Office of Supplemental Security Income
   Altmeyer Building - Room 545
   6401 Security Boulevard
   Baltimore, MD 20235
   (401)965-3424
   1-800-772-1213
   1-800-325-0781 (TDD)

SSA provides information on Supplemental Security Income (SSI), Social Security Disability Insurance (SSDI), Medicare, Medicaid (and Title XIX, the medical component to Medicaid), energy and food assistance. It also provides information on completing and submitting a Plan for Achieving Self-Sufficiency (PASS).

3. Center for Independence and Access State Department of Mental Retardation State Division of Rehabilitation Services Office of Protection and Advocacy: for advocacy; accessibility; local program information for job training, recreation, housing, and education; and protection against neglect or abuse.

Each town or city should have a listing of these organizations in the front of the phone book for Community Service telephone numbers.

4. Commission on Accreditation for Rehabilitation Facilities
    101 North Wilmot Road, Suite 500
    Tucson, AR 85711
    (602)748-1212 (voice/TDD)

CARF sets the standards and accredits rehabilitation programs nationwide that provide quality services.

5. U.S. Department of Justice
   Civil Rights Division
   Coordination and Review Section
   P.O. Box 66118
   Washington, DC 20035-6118
   (202)514-0301 (voice)
   (202)514-0381 (TDD)

The U.S. Department of Justice provides information or referrals for more information regarding the Americans with Disabilities Act; individual rights and specifics to archectural and procedural accomodations for businesses and organizations.

6. International Headquarters Special Olympics
   1350 New York Avenue, Suite 500
   Washington, DC. 20005
   (202)628-3630

Provides information regarding sports, events, and volunteering in local areas.

7. United Cerbral Palsy
   1660 L Street. NW, Suite 700
   Washington, DC 20036-5602
   1-800-USA-5UCP

Provides information, publications, referral resources, and advocacy. Memberships are welcome.

8. Autism Society of America
   7910 Woodmont Ave., Suite 650
   Bethesda, MD 20814-3015
   (301)657-0881

Provides information, publications, referral resources, and advocacy. Memberships are welcome.

9. The ARC, (Association for Retarded Citizens)
   National Headquarters
   500 East Border- Suite 300
   Arlington, TX 76010
   (817)261-6003

Provides information, publications, referral resources, and advocacy. Memberships are welcome.

10. National Down Syndrome Society
    666 Broadway - Suite 810
    New York, NY 10012
    (212)460-9330

Provides information, publications, referral resources, and advocacy. Memberships are welcome.

11. National Parents Network on Disabilities
    1600 Prince Street - Suite 115
    Alexandria, VA 22314
    (703)836-1232

Provides information, publications, referral resources, and advocacy. Memberships are welcome.

Always contact the national organization that serves to advocate for a particular disorder.

APPENDIX

REFERENCES

1. *AAMR. Mental Retardation: Definition, Classification, and Systems of Supports,* 9th Edition, Washington, DC, American Association on Mental Retardation, 1992.

2. Grossman, H. *Classification in Mental Retardation,* Washington, DC, American Association on Mental Deficiency, Grossman et al, 1983.

3. Smull, M., Harrison, S., *Supporting People with Severe Reputations in the Community,* National Association of State Directors of Developmental Disabilities Services, Inc., Alexandria,VA, 1992.

4. Gertz, J. and Bregman, J., MD, *Autism, A Practical Guide For those Who Help Others,* Continuum Publishing Co., New York, NY, 1990.

5. U.S. Department of Justice, *Americans with Disabilities Act Statutory Deadlines,* Washington, DC, 1990.

6. U.S. Equal Employment Opportunity Commission, *The Americans with Disabilities Act,* Washington, DC, 1992.

7. Dept. of Social Services, *Red Book on Work Incentives, A Summary Guide to Social Security and Supplemental Income Work Incentives for People with Disabilities,* Dept. of Health and Human Services, Baltimore, MD, 1992.

FURTHER READING

1. Unsworth, Tim, *The Lambs of Libertyville, A Working Community of Retarded Adults*, Chicago, Contemporary Books, 1990.

2. Greenfield, Josh, *A Child Called Noah*, New York, Holt, Rinehart and Winston, 1972.

3. McClurg, Eunice, *Your Down Syndrome Child,* New York, Doubleday and Co., Inc., 1986.

4. Spiegle, Jan A. and Richard A. van den Pol, *Making Changes: Family Voices on Liviing with Disabilities,* Univ. Montana, 1993.

5.Greenstein, Ph.D., *Backyards and Butterflies, Ways to Include Children with Disabilities in Outdoor Activities,* Cornell Univ.,1995.

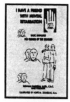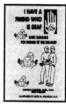